The Galveston Diet Solution

Proven Methods for Reducing Inflammation, Boosting Metabolism, and Balancing Hormones

B. TERZA

© [2024] B. TERZA. All rights reserved.

No part of this publication may be reproduced, distributed, or transmitted in any form or by any means, including photocopying, recording, or other electronic or mechanical methods, without the prior written permission of the author, except in the case of brief quotations embodied in reviews and certain noncommercial uses permitted by copyright law.

The Galveston Diet Solution

Table of Contents

B. TERZA

The Galveston Diet Solution

INTRODUCTION

In a world full of wellness and health fads, the Galveston Diet stands out like a beacon of light. It is specifically developed for women navigating the complexities of metabolic health, hormonal transitions, and midlife. This diet comprises a thorough strategy as well as a meal plan aimed at reducing inflammation, improving metabolism, and restoring hormone balance. Throughout this book, you will discover that the Galveston Diet is more than simply a diet; it is a way of life founded on community, empowerment, and science.

Summary of Diet in Galveston

Fundamentally, the Galveston Diet is designed to address the unique health concerns that women have, particularly during and after menopause. It promotes the concepts of macronutrient tracking, anti-inflammatory eating, and intermittent fasting. This diet recognizes that as women age, their bodies experience significant hormonal changes that might affect their weight, energy levels, and overall health. The Galveston Diet provides you with the information and resources you need to effectively navigate these changes, providing a long-term path to achieving your health goals.

One of the Galveston Diet's core pillars is intermittent fasting, which prioritizes timing of meals above content. Numerous studies have shown that this approach can reduce inflammation, improve metabolism, and aid in weight loss. When you limit your eating to specific times of day, your body may enter a fasting condition. This can aid in cellular repair, boost insulin sensitivity, and promote fat loss.

The anti-inflammatory dietary strategy helps to lower inflammatory markers associated with a variety of chronic illnesses by encouraging the eating of substantial, nutrient-dense foods low in sugar and processed carbs. This nutritional approach focuses largely on fruits and vegetables, as well as meals high in healthy fats such as avocados and almonds. The emphasis on whole, unprocessed foods is congruent with recent nutritional science discoveries, which are beginning to support the notion that diet has a significant impact on inflammation and health outcomes.

Dr. Mary Claire Haver's History and Purpose

Dr. Mary Claire Haver, a board-certified OB/GYN who is dedicated about helping women to enjoy their health during the often-stressful transition to menopause, is the driving force behind the Galveston Diet. Many women who had similar challenges may identify with Dr. Haver's personal struggles with weight control and hormone imbalance at the start of her journey. Her clinical experience revealed a significant paucity of treatments specifically geared for midlife women.

Dr. Haver's practice allowed her to see the effects of hormonal swings on women's bodies and lives firsthand. The lack of effective solutions that took into account the specific biological changes that many of her patients were experiencing left them unsatisfied. This revelation inspired her to create a comprehensive, scientifically supported program that helps women to reclaim their health and vigor while also addressing weight control.

Dr. Haver's approach reflects her commitment to community involvement and education. Her goal is to build a supportive network where women can share their experiences and learn from one another, so removing the stigma connected with midlife health difficulties. Her goal is realized in this book, which provides readers with practical tools and ideas for improving their health.

The importance of managing inflammation, metabolism, and hormonal changes

Understanding how hormones, inflammation, and metabolism interact is critical for women seeking to optimize their health during their middle years. Many women experience a variety of symptoms throughout menopause, including mood swings, fatigue, weight gain, and metabolic slowdowns, as a result of variations in estrogen and progesterone levels. These changes may make it more difficult to maintain a healthy weight and a high level of energy.

These problems are frequently caused by a hormone imbalance. For example, a decrease in estrogen levels may result in an increase in visceral fat, which has been related to an increased risk of chronic illnesses such as diabetes and heart disease. Furthermore, hormone fluctuations can affect metabolism by altering how the body breaks down carbohydrates and lipids, making weight management more difficult.

Chronic inflammation is another major factor that has been linked to a variety of health issues, including diabetes, obesity, and cardiovascular disease. Environmental causes, poor food, stress, and sleep deprivation can all cause inflammation. Women can reduce their risk of getting these diseases and improve their overall health by adopting an anti-inflammatory diet and lifestyle.

Incorporating ways to boost metabolism is equally vital. Hormonal balance, physical activity, and muscle mass are among the elements that influence metabolic health. The Galveston Diet provides actionable steps to optimize metabolic function, enabling women to maintain a healthy weight and energy level.

Objectives of the Book

With the guidance of this book, you should be able to deal with the unique health challenges that occur with middle age. Understanding the science behind the Galveston Diet, including its effects on inflammation, metabolism, and hormones, will allow you to make informed decisions that align with your health goals.

The Galveston Diet Solution

Empowerment via Knowledge: The initial goal is to provide a thorough understanding of the Galveston Diet's fundamental concepts. Because knowledge is power, learning about how your body works can help you make better health decisions.

Useful Strategies and Skills for Success: This book contains a wealth of practical techniques and skills that you can easily apply into your daily practice. This book seeks to make the Galveston Diet more approachable and attainable by providing meal planning help, delicious recipes, and fitness options.

Creating a Community of Support: Finally, we will highlight the importance of community and support. Getting involved with others who are on a similar journey can inspire, hold individuals accountable, and provide support. We'll look into how to connect with other Galveston Diet followers and create a network of support.

As you begin The Galveston Diet Solution, remember that this is a journey to reclaim your health, vitality, and confidence during a life-changing period, not just to lose weight. The techniques and tools provided here are intended to help you become a better, more content version of yourself. Let us embrace the power of information, community, and constructive change as we embark on this journey!

(SECTION 1:)

Understanding Hormones, Metabolism, and Inflammation

In the pursuit of health and well-being, particularly in middle age, it is critical to understand the intricate relationships between inflammation, metabolism, and hormones. These three characteristics interact in ways that have the potential to significantly impact a woman's overall well-being, energy, and health. This section will look at the science behind these notions, as well as their application and practical managerial tactics for promoting wellbeing.

1. The Inflammation Science

What is inflammation?

The body's immune system responds to damage, disease, or harmful stimuli by inducing inflammation. It is a defensive response to aid in healing, characterized by redness, heat, swelling, and discomfort. There are two basic types of inflammation: acute and chronic.

Acute inflammation is a short-term reaction to an injury or infection. It typically goes away as the body recovers and rebalances.

Chronic inflammation, on the other hand, is a long-term reaction that can last months or years. It frequently occurs when the immune system continues to react to what it perceives as a threat, causing tissue damage and exacerbating a variety of conditions, including diabetes, heart disease, and arthritis.

The Impact of Chronic Inflammation on Health

Chronic inflammation is increasingly being identified as a main cause of a wide range of health disorders. It has been associated with autoimmune diseases, metabolic syndrome, and obesity. Persistent inflammation increases the risk of serious health problems by triggering a cascade of metabolic events that disrupt normal cellular activities.

According to studies, chronic inflammation may play an important role in the aging process. Increased levels of inflammatory markers, or "inflammaging," may occur in our bodies as we age, potentially hastening the onset of age-related illnesses.

Menopause-related hormonal changes in women may exacerbate inflammation, increasing the risk of diseases such as osteoporosis and cardiovascular disease.
Vaginalista
). Recognizing and treating chronic inflammation is critical for women in their midlife, especially when it comes to maintaining health and avoiding sickness.

The Impact of Inflammation on Women During Menopause

Women going through menopause have a drop in progesterone and estrogen, both of which play significant roles in inflammation management. Reduced levels of these hormones may lead to increased levels of inflammatory cytokines, which can cause hot flashes, mood swings, and weight gain, among other menopausal symptoms.

According to research, women in menopause may be more prone to long-term inflammatory illnesses. For example, inflammatory processes caused by hormonal variations raise the risk of cardiovascular disease in postmenopausal women.

Understanding how inflammation impacts health during menopause is critical for developing strategies that effectively manage symptoms and improve overall well-being. Women can lower inflammation and improve their quality of life by adopting an anti-inflammatory lifestyle that includes regular exercise, nutritious food, and stress management.

2. A description of metabolism

Knowing How Metabolism Alters as We Age

Metabolism is the intricate set of metabolic processes that convert food into energy. There are two main steps involved:

Catabolism releases energy by breaking down molecules.

Anabolism is the process by which energy is used to construct proteins, nucleic acids, and other cellular components.

Numerous factors influence metabolism, including hormone levels, age, gender, and inheritance. Women's metabolic rates drop with age for a variety of causes, including:

Muscle mass loss occurs because muscle tissue burns more calories than fat during rest. Sarcopenia, or the loss of muscle mass with age, is frequent in women, especially after menopause. This causes a slower metabolic rate.

Hormonal Changes: Hormonal variations, such as those in progesterone and estrogen, may affect metabolism. For example, after menopause, reduced estrogen levels may result in increased fat storage and slower metabolism.

Reduced Physical exercise: As people get older, they tend to participate in less physical exercise, which can exacerbate weight gain and metabolic slowing.

Women who want to maintain a healthy weight and improve their metabolism as they age must understand these changes.

Hormonal Fluctuations' Impact on Metabolism

Hormones are vital for regulating metabolism. Insulin, progesterone, and estrogen are especially important for women:

Estrogen: This hormone regulates fat distribution and metabolism. Low estrogen levels can lead to increased fat buildup, particularly in the abdomen.

Progesterone: This hormone affects metabolism and hunger. Variations in body composition and desires might lead to changes.

The hormone insulin is required for the metabolism of glucose. Insulin resistance increases with age, which can lead to weight gain and an increased risk of developing type 2 diabetes.

To mitigate the effects of hormonal fluctuations on metabolism, women can adopt lifestyle measures such as frequent exercise, balanced nutrition, and stress management approaches.

Important Metabolic Processes Related to Weight Control

The following metabolic pathways are very crucial for regulating weight:

Your basal metabolic rate, or BMR, is the number of calories required by your body at rest to support vital physiological activities. Losing weight as we age may become more challenging if our BMR decreases.

The energy required for nutritional digestion, absorption, and metabolism is referred to as the Thermic Effect of Food (TEF). Certain foods, particularly those high in protein, can increase TEF, which aids in weight management.

Physical Activity: Being physically active on a daily basis increases total energy expenditure, making it crucial for weight management. Resistance exercise has two benefits: it helps to maintain muscle mass and increases metabolism.

Women can optimize their metabolism and promote healthy weight control by making informed decisions based on their understanding of these metabolic processes.

3. Hormone Balance: The Key to Good Health

An overview of the roles of hormones.

Hormones are chemical messengers that regulate a variety of bodily activities, including mood, metabolism, and reproduction. Important hormones for females include:

Estrogen: This hormone is necessary for reproductive health and controlling the menstrual cycle. It also has an impact on cardiovascular and mental health, as well as bone health.

Progesterone: This hormone helps regulate the menstrual cycle and prepares the body for pregnancy. It also has mood-calming properties.

Testosterone: Although commonly associated with men, women can also produce this hormone, which is required for libido, energy levels, and muscular strength.

Insulin is a hormone that regulates fat accumulation and blood glucose levels. Insulin sensitivity is needed for proper metabolism.

Cortisol: Also known as the stress hormone, cortisol regulates immune responses and metabolism. Prolonged stress can elevate cortisol levels, compromising one's health and weight.

Typical women's hormonal imbalances

Hormonal imbalances can manifest in a variety of ways and at different stages of life. Common female hormonal abnormalities include:

Estrogen Dominance: Symptoms such as bloating, mood changes, and weight gain are typically caused by estrogen levels that are significantly higher than progesterone.

Low progesterone: This can cause mood swings, irregular menstrual cycles, and difficulty sleeping.

Insulin Resistance: This disorder, which is usually associated with weight gain and the metabolic syndrome, is caused by cells that are less responsive to insulin, resulting in elevated blood sugar levels.

Adrenal Fatigue: Prolonged stress can produce dysregulation of the cortisol production system, resulting in weight gain, hunger, and weariness.

It is critical to discover these irregularities in order to develop strategies that successfully balance hormones and improve overall health.

Methods to Reach Hormone Equilibrium

A multimodal strategy comprising food modifications, stress reduction, and lifestyle changes is required to establish hormonal equilibrium.

Balanced Diet: Consuming nutrient-dense foods can aid in hormonal equilibrium. To obtain the necessary vitamins and minerals, focus on lean meats, a variety of fruits and vegetables, and healthy fats such as nuts and avocados.

Regular exercise, particularly cardiovascular and strength training, can aid with weight management, metabolism, and hormone balance.

Stress management: Using stress-reduction techniques such as yoga, meditation, or mindfulness can help lower cortisol levels and maintain hormonal balance.

Sleep hygiene: Getting adequate sleep is vital for hormone regulation. To promote overall health, strive for 7-9 hours of restful sleep each night.

Hydration: Staying well hydrated helps hormonal balance and metabolic functioning. Make sure you're drinking plenty of water all day.

Regular check-ups: By monitoring hormone levels, frequent medical checks can detect anomalies early and give appropriate treatment.

Implementing these strategies can help women enhance their hormonal health while also increasing their vitality and well-being.

(SECTION 2:)

The foundation of the Galveston Diet

The Galveston Diet Solution is built on three essential concepts: anti-inflammatory foods, macronutrient tracking, and intermittent fasting. It offers a complete approach to health and wellness. These pillars, which address inflammation, balance hormones, and improve metabolism, aim to empower women—particularly those in their midlife—to take responsibility of their health.

4. Fundamental Concepts of the Galveston Diet

Overview of the Three Pillars.

The Galveston Diet is founded on the belief that our lifestyle and dietary choices have a significant impact on our health. This diet concept is built upon three main ideas:

Intermittent fasting is a successful method that focuses on both when and what you eat. It entails alternating periods of eating and fasting, which can improve insulin sensitivity and reduce inflammation.

Anti-inflammatory meals: This notion emphasizes the importance of eating well-balanced, nutrient-dense meals that enhance overall health and minimize inflammation. Consuming a variety of anti-inflammatory foods can make you feel better and reduce your risk of acquiring chronic illnesses.

Tracking macronutrients: Maintaining hormonal balance and metabolic health necessitates a grasp of protein, fat, and carbohydrate ratios. This notion encourages attentive eating and helps women make informed food choices.

How These Ideas Support Metabolic Processes and Hormonal Health

Each of these principles is linked to the others and is critical to metabolic and hormonal health:

Intermittent fasting provides two important benefits: weight loss and enhanced insulin sensitivity. According to research, irregular fasting can reduce inflammation and insulin levels, both of which are necessary for hormone balance and a healthy weight.

Anti-inflammatory foods provide the body with the nutrients it requires to function optimally. Foods high in antioxidants, vitamins, and omega-3 fatty acids improve immunity and can reduce the inflammatory response caused by hormonal fluctuations.

Women can tailor their diets to their specific needs by employing macronutrient tracking. By balancing protein, fats, and carbohydrates, women can maintain stable energy levels, muscle mass, and hormonal balance.

When combined, these ideas form a solid foundation for achieving health goals, increasing energy, and improving quality of life.

5. Timing is important for intermittent fasting.

An explanation for intermittent fasting.

Intermittent fasting (IF) is a lifestyle that alternates between eating and fasting periods. The most prominent techniques include:

16/8 Method: Eat within an 8-hour window following 16 hours of fasting, frequently skipping breakfast.
Diet 5:2: Eat normally five days a week and reduce your calorie intake (to 500-600 calories) on the two non-consecutive days.
Alternate-Day Fasting: Swap days when you eat normally with days when you fast or consume extremely little calories.
These strategies aid in weight loss and metabolic health by putting the body into ketosis, a state in which it burns fat for energy.

Advantages of Metabolism and Inflammation

Studies show that intermittent fasting can improve metabolic health and significantly reduce inflammation. Among the major benefits are:

Reduced Inflammatory Markers: It has been shown that IF reduces pro-inflammatory cytokine levels, which are linked to chronic inflammation and diseases such as arthritis and heart disease.

Improved Insulin Sensitivity: Intermittent fasting increases insulin sensitivity, which helps the body use glucose more efficiently and may help prevent type 2 diabetes.

Weight Loss and Fat Loss: IF can aid in weight loss, particularly visceral fat, which is linked to metabolic diseases, by creating a calorie deficit and encouraging fat oxidation.

Hormonal Regulation: Fasting can increase levels of growth hormone, which aids in fat loss and muscle maintenance, as well as hormones such as norepinephrine, which promote fat burning.

Helpful Tips for Starting and Maintaining Intermittent Fasting

Starting intermittent fasting can be simple and enjoyable. The following practical advice can help you start and maintain this lifestyle:

Choose a Fasting Approach That Works for You: Experiment with various fasting techniques to see which one best suit your preferences and way of life. Choose a strategy that appears doable, such as the 5:2 diet or the 16/8 technique.

Stay Hydrated: Drink plenty of water during fasting to lessen hunger and improve overall health. Black coffee with no extra sugar and herbal teas may also be good options.

Emphasis on Nutrient-Dense Foods: When breaking your fast, focus on entire, nutrient-dense foods such fruits and vegetables, lean meats, and healthy fats.

Listen to Your Body: Monitor how fasting impacts your body's reactions. If you experience extreme hunger or exhaustion, think about modifying your fasting window or consulting a medical expert.

Be Consistent: Reliability is essential for any lifestyle modification. To aid in your body's adaptation, try to stick to your fasting regimen, especially on the weekends.

Find Support: Look for a friend who is interested in intermittent fasting or join a community. Talking about your experiences helps keep you accountable and inspired.

You can realize the many advantages of intermittent fasting and establish the framework for long-term health gains by putting these tips into practice.

6. Choosing Foods That Reduce Inflammation

Fruits, vegetables, and healthy fats are foods to appreciate.

Choosing anti-inflammatory foods that nourish the body and fight inflammation is the cornerstone of the Galveston Diet. Include the following important groups in your diet:

Nuts (walnuts, almonds), seeds (chia seeds, flaxseeds), and fatty fish (salmon, mackerel) are good sources of omega-3 fatty acids. It is well documented that these fats decrease inflammation and support heart health.

Fruits and Vegetables: Choose a range of bright fruits and vegetables as they are high in phytonutrients and antioxidants. Broccoli, peppers, berries, and leafy greens are especially beneficial for decreasing inflammation.

Whole Grains: Because whole grains are high in fiber and beneficial for your gut, choose ones like quinoa, brown rice, and oats.

Legumes: Chickpeas, lentils, and beans are fantastic sources of fiber and plant-based protein that can be included in a balanced diet.

Items to Steer Clear of: Sugars, processed meals, and unhealthy fats

In addition to focusing meals that reduce inflammation, it's vital to steer clear of items that raise inflammation:
Processed Foods: Foods high in refined carbohydrates, trans fats, and additives can cause inflammation in the body. Fast food, sugary snacks, and premade meals come into this group.

Sugary Drinks: Because they are associated with increased inflammation, sodas and other sweetened beverages should be minimized or eliminated from your diet.

Consumption of red and processed meats has been associated to increased inflammation levels. Instead, select lean protein sources including fish, chicken, and plant-based proteins.

Example menus emphasizing anti-inflammatory options.

This is an example meal plan that focuses on anti-inflammatory foods to demonstrate how to incorporate these principles into your daily routine:

For Breakfast:

Mixed berries and chia seeds sprinkled over Greek yogurt.
A little handful of walnuts to gain healthy fats.
Lunch:

Quinoa salad with cucumber, spinach, cherry tomatoes, and a lemon juice-olive oil vinaigrette.
Carrot and celery stick with hummus on the side.
Snack:

Almond butter spread over sliced apples.
Dinners are

Herb-seasoned baked fish is served with sweet potato wedges and steamed broccoli.
Dessert:

Dark chocolate containing at least 70% cacao or a small bowl of mixed fruit. Drinking lots of water.

Throughout the day, drink as much water and herbal tea as you want.
By following these guidelines and focusing on anti-inflammatory foods, you can create a balanced and fulfilling diet that will help you accomplish your health goals.

In summary:

The Galveston Diet Framework takes a comprehensive approach to health and well-being, addressing key areas like as inflammation, metabolism, and hormonal balance. Learning the core elements of the Galveston Diet, including as intermittent fasting, anti-inflammatory foods, and macronutrient tracking, will help you improve your health and energy levels. In addition to empowering women to make informed dietary choices, this technique promotes a sustainable lifestyle that may have long-term benefits. If you have the necessary information and resources, you can begin your journey to better health and a more active lifestyle.

CALL TO ACTION

Thank you for reading!

I'd like to personally thank you for taking the time to read my work. I really appreciate your time and effort, and I hope this book has provided you with valuable success tools and insights.

Your feedback is really useful to me as I grow as a writer. I would love to hear your feedback, whether positive or negative, so that I may develop and make future works even more useful and fascinating.

I humbly request that you offer an honest evaluation if you found this book worthwhile or if you believe anything may be improved. Your counsel will help me not only improve, but also become a better person.

Thank you again for your support, and I look forward to hearing from you!

SINCERLY

(SECTION 3:)

Putting Galveston Diet into Practice

The Galveston Diet Solution is a lifestyle movement that empowers women to take responsibility of their health, not just a set of dietary guidelines. You may adopt this diet into your daily routine in a sustainable way if you know how to use it correctly. This section will go over how to create a personalized meal plan, why exercise is essential, and what lifestyle changes are required to help you stay to your diet.

7. Creating a Customized Meal Plan

Advice on Meal Planning and Preparation

Creating a personalized food plan is one of the most effective ways to follow the Galveston Diet. Preparing your meals allows you to stay stocked with nutritious options while also saving time and reducing stress. The actions below will help you:

The Galveston Diet Solution

Before you start meal planning, identify what your personal wellness and health goals are. Do you want to boost your energy, reduce inflammation, or lose weight? Setting specific goals will help influence your food strategy.

Select Your Fasting Window: Plan your meals based on the intermittent fasting approach you've chosen (16/8, 5:2). Meal planning throughout this time period can help you keep to your diet more readily.

Plan Balanced Meals: Every meal should include anti-inflammatory foods, healthy fats, lean meats, and fiber-rich carbohydrates, as recommended by the Galveston Diet. A variety of textures and colors on your plate will ensure that you get a wide range of nutrients.

Batch Cooking: Make large quantities of items that can be easily reheated throughout the week. Casseroles, stews, and soups are great options. Try making grains in big quantities, such as brown rice or quinoa, to use as a base for other recipes.

Use Storage Containers: To keep your food organized and fresh, invest in high-quality meal prep containers. This allows you to control portion amounts and makes it easy to take meals on the go.

Advice for Galveston Diet Shopping

Grocery shopping is an essential part of the Galveston Diet. Here are some tips to ensure that your shopping trips are productive and successful:

Make a shopping list based on your meal plan. Follow this list to avoid impulsive purchases, especially when it comes to processed foods and sugary snacks.

Shop the Perimeter: Whole foods, fresh produce, and proteins are typically found on the grocery store's perimeter, so focus your shopping there. Avoid the inner aisles because they are often filled with processed and unhealthy foods.

Read Labels: Practice reading the labels on food products. Look for products that are low in added sugars, fats, and ingredients.

Whenever possible, buy in bulk staples like legumes, nuts, seeds, and whole grains. This can help you save money while also ensuring you always have healthy options available.

Consider seasonal products: Buying fruits and vegetables in season ensures that you are getting the freshest product possible while also supporting your community's farmers. These options taste better and are often more cost-effective.

Simple Recipes and Sample Shopping Lists

To make grocery shopping easier, here is a sample Galveston Diet shopping list, as well as several quick and easy meals.

Example of a shopping list.

Proteins:

Fish that is heavy in fat, like mackerel, or salmon
Breast of chicken.
Eggs
Tofu or tempeh (for plant-based alternatives)
Good Fats:

Avocado or olive oil
Nuts, such as walnuts and almonds
Seeds (such as flaxseed and chia)
Produce and Fruits:

Berries (strawberries, blueberries, etc.)
leafy greens, such as kale and spinach
cruciferous foods, such as cauliflower and broccoli
Butternut squash or sweet potatoes
Complete Grains:

Quinoa
Grains of brown rice
oats
Legumes:

Dried or canned beans (like lentils and black beans)
Simple Recipes:

Pain Relief Quinoa Salad

Components:

1 cup of cooked quinoa.

Half cup of cherry tomatoes.

One sliced cucumber.

1 cup of finely chopped spinach.

1/4 cup feta cheese (optional).

Two teaspoons olive oil

One lemon's juice

To taste, season with salt and pepper.

Guidelines:

In a large bowl, combine the cooked quinoa, tomatoes, cucumbers, spinach, and feta cheese. Season with salt and pepper after drizzling in lemon juice and olive oil. To mix, toss.

Salmon baked in pan with roasted vegetables.

Components:

Two fillets of salmon

One cup of broccoli florets

1 cup diced sweet potatoes

Two teaspoons olive oil

Herbs (such as thyme and rosemary) and salt

Guidelines:

Set the oven temperature to 400 degrees Fahrenheit (200 degrees Celsius). Place the salmon on a baking sheet and top it with the sweet potato and broccoli. Drizzle in olive oil and season with herbs, salt, and pepper. Bake for 20-25 minutes, or until the salmon is fully cooked and the vegetables are tender.

Pudding containing Chia seeds

Components:

Half a cup almond milk (or any other type of milk)
Three tsp of chia seeds
1 tablespoon maple syrup or honey (optional)
Fresh fruit to garnish

Guidelines:

Combine the sweetener, chia seeds, and almond milk in a bowl. After giving it a good stir, chill for at least four hours or overnight. Before serving, place a fresh fruit on top.

Making nutritious meals will become pleasurable and manageable if you incorporate these shopping lists, recipes, and advice into your daily routine.

8. Including Exercise and Making Lifestyle Adjustments

Exercise's Significance in the Galveston Diet

Even while the Galveston Diet has a strong emphasis on eating, exercise is also necessary to get the best possible health and wellbeing. Exercising is essential for:

Increasing Metabolism: Engaging in regular physical activity can raise your resting metabolic rate, which will increase your calorie burn. This is especially crucial since as people age, their metabolisms tend to slow down.

Reducing Inflammation: Studies have demonstrated that regular exercise reduces the body's inflammatory responses. Exercises that can help achieve this goal include resistance training, walking, and running.

Boosting Energy and Mood: Engaging in physical exercise releases endorphins, which have the ability to elevate mood and lessen depressive and anxious sensations. Increased energy levels throughout the day might also be a result of a regular workout program.

Exercises Suggested for Various Fitness Levels

The Galveston Diet Solution

The beauty of the Galveston Diet is that it can be matched with many types of activity, independent of your fitness level. The following suggestions are provided:

For Novices:

Walking: Aim for five days a week of vigorous walking, starting at 20 to 30 minutes each. This low-impact workout is simple to add into your everyday routine and is fantastic for improving cardiovascular health.

Bodyweight Exercises: You don't need any special equipment to perform easy exercises like push-ups, squats, and lunges at home. Begin by performing 1-2 sets of 8–12 repetitions.

For Intermediate:

Strength Training: Include resistance training at least two to three times a week by utilizing resistance bands or free weights. Perform 2-3 sets of 8–10 repetitions, focusing on your main muscle groups.

Yoga and Pilates: These exercises lessen stress levels while boosting strength, flexibility, and balance. Try to attend 1-2 lessons each week.

For Expert:

High-Intensity Interval Training (HIIT): This style of training mixes brief bursts of intensive activity with rest intervals. HIIT is a useful approach for enhancing cardiovascular fitness and burning fat.

Running or Cycling: Try to engage in at least 150 minutes a week of moderate-intensity aerobic activity if you favor endurance sports.

Changes in Lifestyle to Encourage Diet Adherence

Aside from diet planning and exercise, you can improve your adherence to the Galveston Diet by making lifestyle changes:

Establish a Routine: Making a daily schedule that includes of mealtimes and exercise will help to reinforce healthy behaviors and facilitate sticking to a diet.

Make Sleep a Priority: Adequate sleep is vital for hormone balance and general well-being. Aim for 7 to 9 hours of sleep per night to assist you achieve your weight loss targets.

Manage Stress: Chronic stress can contribute to hormone imbalances and weight gain. Think about adding mindfulness exercises into your everyday routine, such as writing, deep breathing, or meditation.

Remain Hydrated: Throughout the day, sipping on lots of water will boost metabolism and lessen sensations of hunger. Try to get in at least 8 glasses a day, or 64 ounces.

Seek Support: Whether it's from friends, family, or internet communities devoted to the Galveston Diet, surround yourself with people who are encouraging. Giving others access to your struggles and experiences can inspire them and hold them accountable.

Part 4: Community Support and Success Stories

Success stories are the potent tales that encourage and inspire others to follow in the footsteps of those who have undergone similar transformations. This also applies to the Galveston Diet. This section will showcase actual life changes brought about by the diet and stress how important community support is to keeping these improvements going. We hope that by sharing these insights and tools, we can empower and inspire you on your journey to better health and well-being.

9. Actual Life Changes

Case studies of people who adopted the Galveston Diet and were successful.

The Galveston Diet has transformed countless lives, and the stories of those who have successfully implemented this method are both encouraging and inspiring. The following are some notable case studies that highlight the incredible changes people have undergone:

Sarah: From Tiredness to Energy.

Sarah, a 42-year-old mother of three, struggled with exhaustion and weight gain after her pregnancies. After learning about the Galveston Diet's emphasis on hormone health and inflammation reduction, she decided to try it. Within the first two weeks of embracing intermittent fasting, she noticed significant changes in her energy levels. She gave up processed foods and sweets in favor of an anti-inflammatory diet high in foods like almonds, leafy greens, and fatty fish. Sarah lost thirty pounds in six months and reported feeling more energized than she had in a long time. Her physician confirmed that her blood tests had improved, indicating better metabolic health and less inflammation.

Jessica: balancing emotions and hormones

After being diagnosed with hormone abnormalities, Jessica, 35, sought a nutritional plan to help her regain control of her health. She identified with the Galveston Diet's emphasis on tracking macronutrients. She lost 25 pounds and experienced less mood swings and anxiety after learning to balance her intake of healthy fats, proteins, and carbs. Jessica started posting updates about her journey on social media, encouraging people going through similar things. Her experience shows how having a solid understanding of macronutrients may have a significant positive influence on one's mental and physical health.

Michael: A Brand-New Beginning

Michael, a 50-year-old with a family history of diabetes and heart disease, was disturbed by his growing cholesterol readings and weight. Following a nutritionist's advice, he went with the Galveston Diet. Michael lost forty pounds, improved his blood sugar and cholesterol, and reduced his body fat by focusing on complete, unprocessed foods and frequent exercise. His narrative emphasizes the significance of changing to a more holistic way of living and demonstrates how a healthy diet can dramatically lower the chance of developing chronic illnesses.

Testimonials Highlighting Better Metabolism, Hormonal Balance, and Decreased Inflammation

The testimonials of individuals who have adopted the Galveston Diet provide witness to their success stories, as they frequently emphasize the same primary advantages: less inflammation, enhanced metabolism, and better hormonal balance. These are some powerful testimonies:

Maria says, "Before starting the Galveston Diet, I was always tired and felt bloated after meals. After a few weeks of intermittent fasting and focusing on anti-inflammatory foods, I noticed my bloating disappeared, and I had so much more energy! I feel like I can keep up with my kids now!"

Lily says, "As a woman in my 40s, I was struggling with weight gain and mood swings. The Galveston Diet taught me about macronutrient tracking and the importance of whole foods. I not only lost weight but also feel more balanced emotionally. I'm so grateful for this diet and the community that supports it."

Tom says, "I had high cholesterol and was facing some serious health risks. Switching to the Galveston Diet was a game-changer for me. I lost weight, my cholesterol levels improved, and I feel healthier than ever. I've even started running again!"

These testimonies demonstrate how the Galveston Diet has given people the means to drastically improve their health. They serve as an example of the beneficial outcomes that can happen when someone adopts a supportive, long-term approach to nutrition.

10. Building a Community of Support

The Community's Function in Sustaining Dietary Changes

Any dietary adjustment that is successful must have the backing of a community. Having a support system of people who have been through the Galveston Diet before can be really beneficial. The following are some explanations on why community support is crucial:

Accountability: You can develop a sense of accountability by discussing your objectives and advancement with others. It motivates you to stick to your dietary adjustments knowing that people are aware of your journey.

Motivation & Encouragement: Getting healthy is not always easy. A supportive community may provide encouragement during hard times, celebrating your triumphs and helping you negotiate hurdles.

Exchange of Information and Resources: Community members can provide insightful advice, scrumptious recipes, and other materials that improve your Galveston Diet experience. You can find fresh success tactics and steer clear of familiar errors by learning from the experiences of others.

Emotional Assistance: Starting a new diet can be a difficult emotional process. Making connections with people who share your journey might help you feel less alone and frustrated by giving you a sense of understanding and belonging.

The Galveston Diet Solution

Resources to Help You Connect with People Traveling Similar Paths

For anyone wishing to establish connections with other Galveston Diet adherents, there are numerous resources at their disposal. Here are a few sensible choices:

Online forums: The Galveston Diet is one of the many diets that are discussed in special areas of websites such as Reddit and health-focused forums. By participating in these forums, you can communicate with a larger community, exchange experiences, and ask questions.

Social Media Groups: Platforms like Facebook and Instagram contain various groups and pages dedicated to the Galveston Diet. These groups frequently exchange success stories, recipes, and motivational hacks. To locate vibrant communities, look for groups using keywords like "Galveston Diet Support Group" or anything similar.

Local Meetups and Workshops: There may be local meetups or workshops centered around the Galveston Diet or related health subjects, depending on where you live. By taking part in these activities, you can meet people who share your interests and exchange personal stories.

Support Systems and Coaching: A few experts provide coaching services that are especially designed for the Galveston Diet. These coaches frequently establish encouraging surroundings for their clients while offering individualized direction and inspiration.

Social media groups, support networks, and online forums

To get the most out of the Galveston Diet, have a look at these particular web resources:

Join Facebook communities: Participate in groups like "Galveston Diet Community" to exchange advice, recipes, and success stories. Talking to other people can provide you more inspiration and wisdom.

Instagram users should follow Galveston Diet accounts. Numerous users contribute their meals, makeovers, and advice, fostering a thriving support and inspiration group.

Reddit: For conversations regarding diet advice, weight loss strategies, and individual experiences, check out the r/loseit or r/Galveston Diet subreddits. These platforms allow you to ask questions and receive advise from people who have followed the program.

YouTube: A lot of diet lovers and health gurus use the platform to share their Galveston Diet experiences. These movies might inspire you and offer useful advice that you can put into practice.

In summary:

The Galveston Diet is a journey that can result in significant changes rather than just a food strategy. Through real-life success stories and testimonies, we see the good impact of reduced inflammation, improved metabolism, and hormonal balance. However, a community's support frequently magnifies success. You may find support, exchange information, and commemorate achievements with people who are traveling a similar path by making connections with them.

Recall that you are not alone as you begin or continue your Galveston Diet adventure. Make use of the tools at your disposal, interact with encouraging groups, and tell your own tale. By working together, we can motivate one another and promote a more energetic, healthy way of living.

As our investigation of the Galveston Diet draws to a close, it's critical to pause and consider the many advantages this dietary strategy has to offer. The Galveston Diet is a complete framework that addresses the particular issues given by hormone shifts, inflammation, and metabolism to enable people—especially women—to regain their health. It is not just another diet craze.

Summary of the Advantages of the Galveston Diet

The three main components of the Galveston Diet are macronutrient tracking, anti-inflammatory foods, and intermittent fasting. All these elements are essential for maintaining a good way of living, especially when menopause is approaching and beyond.

Intermittent Fasting: This method promotes a controlled eating schedule that gives the body time to recuperate in between meals. There is ample evidence to support the benefits of intermittent fasting, which include increased fat reduction, increased insulin sensitivity, and decreased inflammation. Fasting is a useful tool for anyone looking to improve their overall health because studies have shown that it can lead to significant improvements in metabolic health.

Inflammatory Foods: The focus is on eating whole, nutrient-dense foods, such as fruits, vegetables, healthy fats, and lean proteins, which give the body the essential nutrients it needs to function at its best. These foods promote metabolic health and hormonal balance in addition to reducing inflammation. Numerous studies have demonstrated the association between a diet high in anti-inflammatory foods and a decreased chance of developing chronic illnesses such as diabetes, heart disease, and several types of cancer.

For efficient weight management, knowledge of the ratios of the macronutrients—proteins, carbs, and fats—is essential. The Galveston Diet encourages satiety and long-term energy levels by enabling people to customize their diets to meet their own needs. This tailored strategy makes sure that dietary decisions support individual health objectives, such as better energy, weight loss, or hormonal balance.

The Galveston Diet offers a comprehensive framework for attaining long-term health advantages by incorporating these principles. People have completely changed their lives, as seen by the testimonies and success stories scattered throughout this book. They have reduced chronic inflammation, found relief from hormone imbalances, and enhanced their general quality of life.

Motivation to Accept Lifestyle Modifications for Long-Term Health

Adopting the Galveston Diet is a commitment to a better lifestyle, not merely a nutritional adjustment. In order to stay motivated and create long-lasting changes, keep the following principles in mind as you set out on this journey:

Prioritize Progress Over Perfection: Recognize that maintaining good health is a lifetime process. Celebrate the little accomplishments along the road, such as tasting a new dish, adhering to your intermittent fasting regimen, or fitting in more exercise during the day. Your efforts to lead a healthier lifestyle are cumulative.

Create a Support System: Be in the company of encouraging people who share your objectives. Interact with Galveston Diet-supporting communities both online and off. Exchanges of experiences and difficulties can yield priceless inspiration and support.

Make Intentional Decisions: Plan meals mindfully. Observe your body's and your mood's reaction to various foods. This awareness can lead to a better understanding of your body's demands and help you make more educated decisions.

Make Self-Care a Priority: Keep in mind that diet is not the only factor in your health journey. Include self-care activities in your daily routine, such as managing your stress, getting enough sleep, and exercising frequently.

The Galveston Diet Solution

Achieving and preserving hormonal balance and general wellbeing depend on these factors 【6†source】 【7†source】 .

Nutrition by Abby Langer.
The field of ion science is always changing. Stay intrigued and informed about new studies and practices that may enhance your experience with the Galveston Diet. You can fine-tune your strategy and discover what works best for you by being flexible.

In the end, the Galveston Diet gives you the ability to take charge of your health by helping you make decisions based on knowledge about what your body requires. The advantages go beyond just losing weight; they also include increased vitality, better hormone balance, decreased inflammation, and a livelier way of living.

As you embark on your journey or make the initial steps toward the Galveston Diet, never forget that change is not only feasible but also attainable. Accept the changes in your way of life, get involved in your community, and share your personal story. We can create a more vibrant and healthier future if we work together.

CALL TO ACTION

Thank you for reading!

I'd like to personally thank you for taking the time to read my work. I really appreciate your time and effort, and I hope this book has provided you with valuable success tools and insights.

Your feedback is really useful to me as I grow as a writer. I would love to hear your feedback, whether positive or negative, so that I may develop and make future works even more useful and fascinating.

I humbly request that you offer an honest evaluation if you found this book worthwhile or if you believe anything may be improved. Your counsel will help me not only improve, but also become a better person.

Thank you again for your support, and I look forward to hearing from you!

SINCERLY

www.ingramcontent.com/pod-product-compliance
Lightning Source LLC
Chambersburg PA
CBHW061738250726
48657CB00002B/994